They Bloom Because of You

Jessica Urlichs is the *Sunday Times*-bestselling author of *Beautiful Chaos* and a poet who lives in New Zealand with her husband and three children. She has written a variety of children's books to help babies and young children navigate their emotions in their early years. Jess's honest and heartfelt poetry about her family and motherhood continue to be a source of guidance for mothers and parents alike around the world to connect, and her online community continues to grow.

They Bloom Because of You

On the Infinite Love,
Growth and Magic of Motherhood

JESSICA URLICHS

PENGUIN LIFE

AN IMPRINT OF

PENGUIN BOOKS

PENGUIN LIFE

UK | USA | Canada | Ireland | Australia
India | New Zealand | South Africa

Penguin Life is part of the Penguin Random House group of companies whose addresses can be found at global.penguinrandomhouse.com

Penguin Random House UK,
One Embassy Gardens, 8 Viaduct Gardens, London SW11 7BW

penguin.co.uk

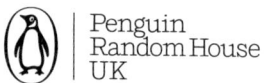

First published 2026

002

Copyright © Jessica Urlichs, 2026

The moral right of the author has been asserted

Penguin Random House values and supports copyright. Copyright fuels creativity, encourages diverse voices, promotes freedom of expression and supports a vibrant culture. Thank you for purchasing an authorized edition of this book and for respecting intellectual property laws by not reproducing, scanning or distributing any part of it by any means without permission. You are supporting authors and enabling Penguin Random House to continue to publish books for everyone. No part of this book may be used or reproduced in any manner for the purpose of training artificial intelligence technologies or systems. In accordance with Article 4(3) of the DSM Directive 2019/790, Penguin Random House expressly reserves this work from the text and data mining exception

Set in 11/14.75pt Garamond MT Std
Typeset by Six Red Marbles UK, Thetford, Norfolk
Printed and bound in Great Britain by Clays Ltd, Elcograf S.p.A.

The authorized representative in the EEA is Penguin Random House Ireland, Morrison Chambers, 32 Nassau Street, Dublin D02 YH68

A CIP catalogue record for this book is available from the British Library

ISBN: 978–0–241–76511–1

Penguin Random House is committed to a sustainable future for our business, our readers and our planet. This book is made from Forest Stewardship Council® certified paper.

For you, always remember – they bloom because of you

Contents

Introduction	5
There Is a Mother Somewhere	7
Where I Begin	10
When a Mother Falls in Love	12
I'll Hold Your Hand	15
To My Midwife	17
Neither You, Nor I	19
What If	20
A Mother's Love	23
Coffee Is Not Enough	24
A Mother's First Steps	26
All I Love	27
Our Chair	29
Mother	31
I See You Now, My Friend	32
You've Changed	35
While the World Sleeps	37
When I Say Motherhood Is Hard . . .	40
The Way She Shines	41
They Say a Partner's Love Has No Limits	42
Borrowed Time	44
The First Year (Again)	46
Texts Between Friends	49
It's All So Simple	52
Thin Skin Fragile Hearts Club	55

Two Things Can Be True	56
The House That Raised Our Family	59
She Is Two	61
Unravelled	63
Playdates	64
My Nightlight Down the Hall	65
A Radical Love	68
Love Near the Chair	71
More Than a Body	73
Heart and Hands	74
Strong Women	75
My Daughter	76
Tiny Days	77
Take Me With You	79
The Spaces Between	81
The Vows I Didn't Write	83
A Mind Like Mine	86
Becoming	89
I Mean Well	90
When the World Feels Too Much	91
To Love a Boy	92
A Love That Doesn't Rest	93
You're Doing It	97
Am I Still Your Baby, Mama?	100
My Middle Child	103
The Friends We Hold Close	105
This Hard Has Been My Happiest	106
Who She Would Have Been	108
When Mummy Was Your Name	110
First Day	112
Be Seeing You	113

There's Something About That Third Child	116
The Mental Load	117
The Mums Who Walk Each Other Home	119
Cracked Open	120
Rested Eyes	121
Missing: Brain	123
A Love Note to My Younger Self	124
Why Are You So Tired?	127
But We Lived	128
I Miss You	129
Tiptoe, Off You Grow	132
The School Gate	133
Today You Turn Six	135
For Grandad	137
I Point Out Every Blossom Tree	138
A Human First	139
You'll Always Be With Me	142
The Current	144
Where Love Lives	145
Boys Will Be Boys	147
When I Tell My Daughter 'I Love You Too'	148
The Song of Motherhood	150
Not Just the Family Dog	152
Three Plus Me	156
The Good Old Days	158
Today You Turn Seven	160
Your Motherhood Lives On	162
Here We Are	163
They Bloom Because of You	164
Acknowledgements	167

Introduction

In motherhood there are seasons we grow through as much as they grow through us. These pages offer a glimpse of the stories they hold, the ache, the love, and the becoming.

There Is a Mother Somewhere

There is a mother somewhere,
whose grown child lives on the other side of the world,
she holds them in her heart because of the distance
between their arms.

There is a mother somewhere,
whose baby won't stop crying,
they want to be held, fed to sleep, they need her so much
and all she wants is a moment alone.

There is a mother somewhere,
whose child may never say the word 'mama',
she's faced unimaginable challenges,
and dreams of that sound often.

There is a mother somewhere,
who has heard the word 'mummy' on repeat,
she's touched out, it's all so loud,
and she's desperate for a moment of silence.

There is a mother somewhere, awake,
tiptoeing out the door of the nursery, her tears not long dried,
she dreams of sleep, she adores her baby
but still thinks back to those carefree days sometimes.

There is a mother somewhere, awake,
who hears tiptoeing down the hallway
because her teenager got in late,
she loves watching them grow,
but she thinks back to the days they were little
and would climb into her bed for cuddles instead.

There is a mother somewhere,
her house is full of noise and mess, lived in and loved.

There is a mother somewhere,
her house is clean and silent, and memories hang on the walls.

There is a mother somewhere,
telling her grandchildren about what their parents were like
when they were little.

There is a mother somewhere,
asking her own mother, what was it like?

It's heartachingly beautiful, and sometimes,
a beautiful heartache.

If she tells you this is incredible, the best thing
she's ever done, believe her.

If she tells you this is hard, the hardest thing
she's ever done, *believe her.*

It's heartachingly beautiful, and sometimes, a beautiful heartache.

THEY BLOOM BECAUSE OF YOU, JESSICA URLICHS

Where I Begin

You made me a mother
and so much more
I became a home
and you opened that door.

My heart took a leap
left my body anew
a wholesome hollow
when we became two.

You took your first breath
as I held my own
the world stood still
as you started to roam.

I've been out of my mind
and I've been in my head
like a hallway of frames
filled with you instead.

And no song sounds as sweet
nor the ocean, nor birds,
as the hum in my memory
of your first words.

See, I can't explain
this weakness and strength
where you begin
and where I end.

My voice became louder
a whisper turned roar
it's hard to imagine
my life before.

Because I'd give you the world
but my heart will have to do
for they're one and the same
now it lives in you.

When a Mother Falls in Love

People will try to tell you about that first moment.
When you fall in love.

And you'll nod, you'll sit there in awe trying to make sense of a feeling that could never be put into words.

Because how do you explain about knowing love but not like this, how it runs through your veins. How with each inhale you'll consume it for ever from this moment forward. That your new home is wherever they are, and theirs is simply you.

How do you explain this pain with a purpose, the one that pulls every ounce of strength from your body. Strength you never knew you had, strength that waited for you.

How do you explain wanting the world to know about this perfect little person you're staring down at, and in the same breath, wanting to protect them from it. That you've never felt so fierce and so vulnerable, that your arms have never felt so important.

How do you explain that those months of growing them would be the beginning of them growing you. How you can be born again, still you and someone new.

How do you explain how it feels as if you've known them for ever. How they find your eyes like it's all they've been searching for.

How do you explain how time will stand still, but never still enough to catch it.

How your legs will wobble in this new role and yet you'll never stand so tall, and how heartbeats have their own language.

That this love has a sense of melancholy, you'll feel everything, it's so big it hurts. It's peaceful and it's terrifying.

A journey where your destination travels alongside you.
A detached piece of yourself that makes you feel whole.
A colour before the bloom.
A type of magic handmade just for us.
Maybe that's why no words could ever do it just.

How do you explain how time will stand still, but never still enough to catch it.

THEY BLOOM BECAUSE OF YOU, JESSICA URLICHS

I'll Hold Your Hand

There will always be days where the world feels tough
So let me remind you that you are enough.

There will always be lows, there will always be highs
So hold my hand, and together we'll fly.

There will always be troubles, but tomorrow is new
So hold my hand, and let me show you.

There will always be darkness, but the sun will still rise
So hold my hand, let your glow be your light.

There will always be sadness, but there's love on the shore
Let it wash over you, hold my hand a bit more.

For each crack in the earth, a star shines above
For each heart that breaks, someone's falling in love.

And for every beginning, there'll be someone you miss
You can hold my hand through it, I'm so glad you exist.

There's pain and there's beauty, there's joy and there's fear
And in each given moment, I'm so happy you're here.

So, when it seems heavy and it's harder to stand
You can lean on me instead, I'll hold your hand.

In each given moment, I'm so happy you're here.

THEY BLOOM BECAUSE OF YOU, JESSICA URLICHS

To My Midwife

I don't know how to thank you
For all that you have done
The way that you move heaven and earth
A hero who's unsung.

The power you have witnessed
How you reminded me
The strength I had within
The beauty that you see.

And all those months you listened
Measured, soothed, and cared
The texts and calls you took
The way that you were there.

It takes someone so special
To do all that you do
To hold each birth close to your heart
And all the heartbreaks too.

And though I felt so vulnerable
In those moments of love and pain
You told me I was strong
Again, and again, and again.

You guided a life into this world
And then you guided another
In all the weeks thereafter
As I became a mother.

And each time I would soften
As you walked through my door
It feels a little strange
That I won't see you any more.

So, I just want to thank you
For this huge part of my life
I'll always remember that day
And I'll always remember my midwife.

Neither You, Nor I

Mama, we haven't done this before,
Neither you, nor I.
We both feel very small,
And these arms don't feel like mine.

It's very hard to focus
And everything is new
But I hear a voice as you pull me in
And my heart knows it is you.

I know that you are tired
Full of worry, love and fear
But only when I'm with you
Do my worries disappear.

So, let's lie here together
Let's take it day by day
Just press my heart against your own
And let it show the way.

Mama, please don't fear these days
For they will pass us by.
We're both brand new,
We haven't done this before.

Neither you, nor I.

What If

What if in the beginning
We told mothers it was okay?
To surrender, give in, hold on, as long
As the night turned into day.

And what if from the start
We supported how a mother feeds?
If she could, or couldn't, or simply chose
To remember her own needs.

And what if we said 'it's normal'
To not always feel so together?
Let's change 'just you wait and see'
To 'it won't be like this for ever'.

And instead of holding the baby
What if we held the mother?
And walked together on this journey
One foot after the other.

And what if we encouraged her
To do whatever felt right?
To soften into her knowing
In the harder parts of night.

And what if we spoke of all the shades
　　The sunsets and the blues?
That her path is hers, and how beautiful it is
　　To find something you didn't lose.

And instead of holding the baby What if we held the mother?

THEY BLOOM BECAUSE OF YOU, JESSICA URLICHS

A Mother's Love

You must have known I loved you,
Before you came to be.
By some divine miracle
You found your way to me.

You must have felt my love for you
Before you could even feel.
You must have heard my call for you
Before you were even real.

And now we lie together
A new familiar gaze.
I promise that I'll never
Be the first to look away.

I've loved you for the longest time
Much longer than it seems.
Before we even met
Because I loved you in my dreams.

Coffee Is Not Enough

Here's to the mums who feed to sleep
Have forgotten to eat
Pick things up with their feet.
Here's to the mums who have a quick shave,
Just of their ankles
No time in the day.
Here's to the mums who quickly walk by
Their furry first baby
Whose tail wags to say hi.
Here's to the mums who think they've done nothing
Being someone's constant
Is more than just something.
Brain is scattered, mismatched like socks
On your worst day
You are still someone's rock.
And here's to the mums who feel they may break
With each little startle
And every night wake.
Tired and tangled, this is no easy feat
But just a reminder:
Please have something to eat.

*On your worst day
You are still
someone's rock.*

THEY BLOOM BECAUSE OF YOU, JESSICA URLICHS

A Mother's First Steps

None of regulating their big emotions while
trying to regulate your own is easy.

No one can tell you how to do this,
no one knows your children like you do,
even on the days you feel like you don't.

This isn't a dress rehearsal, there is no main act,
no true measurable goals,
only the moment before you.

You can't hold on to everything you did or didn't do,
there are no receipts or score cards, no winning
or losing, just being, and feeling, and connecting,

and disconnecting
and love bursting forth
and numbness in between it all,
and trying,
and trying,
and trying again.

All I Love

I love that I get to hold you
And swoop in when you call
Hold myself out like a blanket
Be your landing when you fall

I love that I'm your safety
That it's my hand you hold
I love how it is my embrace
That weaves your pain to gold

I love that on the longest nights
As you drift off to my smell
My heavy head tomorrow
Is all on which to dwell

I love that I'm that place
For your worries and your fears
My heartbeat in a shell
Like an ocean to your ears

I love that in the morning
Even in the early rise
My face over the cot
Is the light behind your eyes

I love these slow and gentle days
How they blend with one another
Always the mother of a baby
And the baby of a mother

But I hurt for all I love
For the mothers who want nothing more
Than to go back to the hard beginnings
That seemed so hard before

My heart is torn for all I love
And so, I hold you close
For those with aching hearts
Who know a mother's love the most.

Our Chair

I know we are here a lot, Mama,
together in this chair
but right now I don't want to be
anywhere but here.

It's warm, and it's familiar,
yet every moment is new;
little building blocks
of the safety that is you.

I won't recall these memories
these nights of you and me,
how when I cry out again, and again
it's your beautiful face I see.

But your soothing will be my song,
your skin will be my home.
This belonging will always live in my heart
even when I'm alone.

Your voice shines through the darkness
as you lift me to your embrace,
my little hands search for you,
as you wipe tears from my face.

One day our nights won't look like this,
one day you'll set me down.
I'll never sleep on you again,
with no chair to be found.

The chair will become your arms,
or the comfort of your smile.
The chair will become your voice on the phone
that I've missed hearing for a while.

So for now, Mama, please hold me close
back and forth together,
I may not remember our chair
but I'll carry these moments for ever.

Mother

You're not just a person
You're a place.
You are someone's home.

I See You Now, My Friend

I wish I could say, 'I see you'
As I think back to before
How I watched you become a mother
But it wasn't you I saw

You shared your announcement photo
Your baby, all brand new
'Welcome to this world' it read
And it should have been for you

I wish I'd held you before the baby
And listened between the lines
Maybe I would have asked again
When you told me you were fine

I wish I'd seen more than the smiles
And realized your tears had dried
And known your sun had become the one
That set in your baby's eyes

And when you said you were tired
I wish I knew what you meant
I nodded, imagining the longest nights
But your body felt broken and bent

I wish I had known that consuming love
And truly celebrated your wins
The privilege of being invited over
As you let the outside in

I wish I had seen the immense change
And not just of your view
That even though you were so in love
At times you felt lonely too

That as magnificent as you seemed
You had your doubts and fears
That a piece of you now lived on your sleeve
And your moods were mapped by theirs

I wish I had listened more closely
The first smiles, first rolls, and feeding
And just how big these achievements were
How you told me these days were fleeting

And when you left the house those times
I wish now that I knew
What was involved, the planning, the effort
and all you had to do

It's not that I wasn't in awe
Of when you became a mother
I just missed the shine in your eyes
As you swayed and stared at each other

I appreciate you so deeply now
As I too feel rearranged
I guess I didn't look hard enough
To see the woman that had changed

As I hold my world, my bones, my heart
I think of you back then
How I watched you become a mother
But I see you now, my friend.

You've Changed

And maybe I have.
I no longer only see myself when I stare in the mirror.
My centre is the soil of what now blooms around me.
I've walked through one hundred lives to finally stand still
I've snapped the stems of my past to grow a new future.
I've travelled to the stars and never left Earth,
screamed in silence, held my own beating heart,
rested with these new familiar bones
and you tell me I have changed.
How kind of you to notice.

My centre is the soil of what now bloom around me.

THEY BLOOM BECAUSE OF YOU, JESSICA URLICHS

While the World Sleeps

For the mother who is awake while everyone sleeps,
it only feels that way because we're all in the same stillness.

There are many of us awake,
pacing, shushing, sitting in our chairs. Wrapped up in them, and
the quiet of the world.

There are many of us awake,
gently holding their little hand to our face as they feed,
gazing at each other, whispering heartbeats.

There are many of us awake,
some still tender from birth. Scooping up their softness with
tears in our eyes. A new and powerful attunement. A lifetime of
knowing each other, in the way only a mother and baby could.

There are many of us awake,
exhausted and in love, tired and tangled. Doubting whether we
are doing this right, while our babies sigh in comfort and
look at us as if we scattered the stars in the sky.

There are many of us awake,
with eyes that open before hearing their cries, with ears that
listen for each puff of their breath, with a body that aches, and
sways, as the sun slowly stretches its arms.

There are many of us awake,
in all this tired magic, holding sunshine in human form while the moon hangs lazily in the sky.

There are many of us awake,
it's 2 a.m. and your baby is sleeping. A moment you won't miss, and yet you will. A memory of when all it took was you, your smell, your presence, your touch.

And suddenly, such a small hour takes up the biggest space in your heart.

Holding sunshine in human form.

THEY BLOOM BECAUSE OF YOU, JESSICA URLICHS

When I Say Motherhood Is Hard . . .

What I mean is, it's not motherhood, it's the mental load.
It's not the baby, it's the broken sleep.
It's not the lack of alone time, it's the lack of a village.
It's not matrescence, it's the not prioritizing maternal mental health.
It's not failing at breastfeeding, it's society's expectations failing me.
It's not the no days off, it's the no hands on.
It's not my postpartum body, it's the pressure to 'bounce back'.
Pregnancy glow to let herself go.
It's being over being undervalued.
I love being a mother, but motherhood is hard,
And maybe it could be easier.

The Way She Shines

I whispered to the stars once
I fear I've lost my glow
I said I missed my sparkle
And they told me what they know.
It takes a mother's strength, they said
To burn brightly all the time
We see the way you sparkle
And the way you share your shine.
But I fear it's not enough
And they simply said to me
Look beyond the glitter night,
And tell me what you see.
It was then I saw a little glow
And it gazed into my eyes
A reflection so familiar
That it caught me by surprise
There's proof your sparkle never left,
You've shared it with someone.
For the moon can only shine, they said
From the brightness of the sun.

They Say a Partner's Love Has No Limits

They say love has no limits
But I don't think that's true
For a last is a limit, and our love is not new.
It's not in the spark, the grand gestures and gold
I think the real treasure is found in the old.
We've watched time stand still, we've changed our pace
Less mystery to uncover, more magic to embrace.
We saw less romance, and more routine,
With fewer fireworks and more fatigue.
But the world fell away as you held my hand
and our love climbed like vines, all over again.
It wasn't all perfect, I wished times away
We'd argue and cut round the bruise of our day.
But we laughed and we loved, we showed up for each other
When all of our firsts became that of another.
You've been my rock, you are my home.
The new was beautiful, but I'd rather be known.
Though a love with no limits may last for ever,
I just want to live all of our lasts together.

It's not in the spark, the grand gestures and gold I think the real treasure is found in the old.

THEY BLOOM BECAUSE OF YOU, JESSICA URLICHS

Borrowed Time

There's an arm of light that reaches in
and splits the room in two.
We're on borrowed time, my love,
here, just me and you.
There's a rocking chair, your sleepy breath,
and little kicking feet.
Borrowed time, my love, a place
the two of us will meet.
There's a hanging moon, heavy with hope,
a cot rail etched with scars.
It's fate I get to know your skin,
under these tired stars.
There's a tiny hand tracing my face,
a clock ticking away.
If our moments were a story
I would bookmark every page.
Tender nights, I'll think of you,
back when you were mine.
For we're on borrowed time, my love,
We're on borrowed time.

It's fate I get to know your skin, under these tired stars.

THEY BLOOM BECAUSE OF YOU, JESSICA URLICHS

The First Year (Again)

It's a little bit different
to the very first time,
all of your firsts
are no longer mine.

No less special,
some lessons still new
Still realizing
all of the things I can do.

I know what's in store
and the hard days do end
I break a bit less
as I've learnt how to bend.

I'm not striving for perfect,
good enough will do
I don't bother with books
I know to read you.

I'm a little less bothered
with the toys and the mess
I know that achievements
mean doing my best.

I do what feels right
with a much louder voice
I guess you stop listening
when you block out the noise.

But I don't know it all,
I'm still caught by surprise,
more tired than ever
with much softer eyes.

My arms are much stronger
as I've carried for years
There are maps on my face
from smiles and tears.

I don't chase the milestones
And I don't count the days
It's much faster now
as I'm split in more ways.

It's more rushed than I'd like,
naps wherever we are
Let us just have a moment —
off we go in the car.

It's busy, I know,
and some days I feel spent
While you are all smiles
and cheeks, and content.

I catch myself wishing
as I watch you grow
I could go back to the start
with what I now know.

But each one of you
has helped me grow tall
In the depths of these seasons,
the whirlwind of it all.

You've given me shape
You've taught me to be
You handed me pieces
To this puzzle of me.

I have done this before.
But I haven't with you
This first year, my darling,
is entirely new.

Texts Between Friends

My friend messaged me after I had a baby, 'How are you?'
it read.
I responded,

'It's harder than I thought, some moments I'm swept up in the beauty of motherhood, others I'm dragging myself around in a coffee-stained dressing gown with unwashed hair.
I know people say to take some time out for me, but in this season of being so needed I don't know how.

I'm more tired than I ever imagined, though I could trace their tiny features for hours, I could watch the way a sneeze crinkles their eyes and takes them by surprise.

But I also feel a little lost at times, yet they are a seed in my bones, and I have never been more found.

Some days I sit in shadows, and others the light fills me up inside and together we grow and grow.
My body aches, from birth, for the girl I once was, for sleep, for their scent. The shower feels like a break, though I always feel hurried.

It makes no sense, does it?

Some days I feel as if I'm not achieving much and yet I am rushed off my feet. Years can pass through these four walls in mere minutes.

My mind is all over the place, I want to press pause and yet I am already in awe of who they're becoming.

We're still figuring this whole thing out together, and yet it's like I've known them for ever. I feel a new type of wholeness, of being complete, but some days I just feel empty,

does this make any sense?

I'd love some time alone, but I am entangled in them, and yet that's how I want it. My heart would be fumbling around in the dark without them. That's another thing I wanted to tell you . . . I've never thought with my heart so much, I've never seen so much with it either.

I'm not ready to have visitors just yet, but I miss you, I really do.

Thanks for checking in.'

But I didn't.
Instead, I told her we were great, my baby was simply a dream, and that we couldn't wait to see her.
Then I hit send.

My heart would be fumbling around in the dark without them.

THEY BLOOM BECAUSE OF YOU, JESSICA URLICHS

It's All So Simple

The last leaf fell from babyhood a while ago,
I've sat in the ceaseless storm of toddlerhood since.
Today you just wanted to play with the water in the sink, wanted
another snack, wanted, wanted.
Wanted me.
I was scrubbing the mud from the carpet that you brought in,
and you screamed at me, and then I cracked.
I became the thunder.
I was flooded with regret as your innocent, alarmed face
looked to me,
seeking solace in my safe embrace.
How wrong it feels to calm your heart when I'm the one who
made it race.
So we sit in a rain dance on the floor.
'I'm sorry,' I whisper.
And you weep some more.
I don't have a lot of time to hold my umbrella when
I'm always holding yours.
But this is what we do.
I stroke your curls.
This is what we do.
I hold you back to wipe your tears and offer a smile.
This is what we do.
We get up, you forgive, you still want to play with the
water in the sink.

I slide over the chair and gently bring you up to the tap, water pours through your fingers and sunshine beams from your face.

How can this be so hard when it's all so simple?

Being your world is everything,
and some days that takes everything.

Being your world is everything, and some days that takes everything.

THEY BLOOM BECAUSE OF YOU, JESSICA URLICHS

Thin Skin Fragile Hearts Club

If you have a heart that easily breaks, I feel like
I know you a little.
You never threw rocks, you kept them buried in your chest.
You dodged ants on the sidewalk, and grieve for
those you don't know.
To float like a feather would be wonderful, but please,
don't change.
It's hard to let others in when your skin is thin, but you must,
Because there are many of us,
who hold up drooping flowers by their chins,
who weep for the birdsong of an empty nest,
whose feet are sore from the shoes of many.
You are lionhearted and beautiful.
I know the ache of being cracked open, but this is
how you shine.
And when the world bares its teeth and darkness falls, it is your
light it needs.
The world needs your light.

Two Things Can Be True

Some days I find it hard
and then I wonder how
there's nowhere else I'd rather be
than where I am right now.

The beauty in these moments
they fill me up with light,
but some days cast a shadow
that follows me into night.

And though this is a dream
I'm tired to the bone.
See, some days I feel lost
though I'm never more at home.

Some of us are in the trenches,
some of us are healing
and no amount of gratefulness
should cancel out a feeling.

Achievements look quite different here:
dishes, meals, a nap.
I know I should be proud of these,
but I'm getting used to that.

I've never felt as important before
in any job, not one.
We carry the world, so of course it is hard,
the hardest I've ever done.

And though it can be loud
and I have to squint to think,
I know that I will miss this
when it's over in a blink.

But it's not about the future
for that we cannot see
it's about the highs and lows of now,
the brutal honesty.

It feels a little easier
when another mum says 'same',
I know I'm not alone
in the beauty and mundane.

I'd never trade this life with them,
of course, neither would you.
But it's okay to talk about it all
Because two things can be true.

And no amount of gratefulness should cancel out a feeling.

THEY BLOOM BECAUSE OF YOU, JESSICA URLICHS

The House That Raised Our Family

Our first house was our first home
Where little spongy hands would roam
It's where your eyes began to search
So mine would follow and find
It's where your little feet would wander
And mine began to guide.
Where memories were made, it's where I changed.
Where we grew, where I became.
Some days a castle or a cave.
The walls would hold us late at night
Then catch the laughter in the morning light
Where the days were long and I knew each nook
Lived in its detail like a story book.
First words, first foods, tantrums and tears
We argued a bit during that first year.
And we painted and decorated, loved and danced
It was small and perfect, we made it ours.
But just like life promises change,
We gathered the memories that we made.
Said goodbye, and were on our way.
Then late one night in our new place
Stars poured through the window onto your face
And there we were

Here we are
The same you and I, and moon, and stars.
I still think of the house that saw us grow
But we are the heartbeat of any home.

She Is Two

She is two
With rose petal eyes
She finds her voice
As I even mine

An exquisite tornado
Turns me into a wreck
Her daisy chain arms
The jewels of my neck

She is fury and thunder,
She is sunshine, and heart
With tiny fists of rage
That move mountains apart

She shows up as she is
Hard not to admire
A whale spout on her head
And a dragon of fire

Stubborn and wilful
Her heart on a quest
For joy and wonder
wildness and mess

Cannot be reasoned with
Keeps me guessing
She's the rise in my chest
My heartache, my blessing

Passion without apology
She'll do it herself
Peace in her love
But not much else

Painstakingly wonderful
Exhausted each day
Wouldn't have her
Any other way.

Unravelled

I give so much of myself
Pieces of me are missing,
I wear your smile like my own
I am a museum of your feelings,
I've put my paintbrush down
To watch you draw instead,
I've sat still for the longest time
I'm learning to walk again,
I carry your heart inside
My sleeve now carries mine,
I love you more than anything
So I told anything goodbye,
The shortest and the longest time
Hand in hand we travelled.
One day I'll look back to see
The beautiful tangle unravelled.

Playdates

I just feel a bit lost / no one prepared me for / we're on bottles now / I've been there too / I have a spare snack / talking about it helps / we should do this more often / I miss you / I miss me / What do I wear? / do what works / need a child-free date / to connect again / to compare less / worry less / oh no, we're fine / I'm a better person / but do you feel lonely sometimes? / do you have a spare nappy? / look at those smiles / I lost my patience / mum of the year / said she wants a different mummy / ballet lesson on Saturday / hormones everywhere / it's my old nipple cream / makes a great lip balm / not enough hours in the / very long days / nap time I think / we should get going / may fall asleep in the car / good luck / thank you / *for putting me back together.*

My Nightlight Down the Hall

Ollie the Owl sits next to my bed.
He's blue, he's always blue.
I know I need to wait for him to be orange. But when I wake up and he's still blue it feels lonely and somehow colder than before.
The room feels so big suddenly, and it feels like
something is missing.
It's my mum.

I used to call out when I was much smaller, but now I just
wander down the hallway,
my cuddly in my hand dragging on the carpet behind me.
I hope they're not mad with me, I do this every night.
I know they'd rather I stay in my own bed. I have a sticker chart
on the fridge, but it's still empty.
She somehow always knows I'm coming before I get there, she's usually sitting up ready, and I'm relieved when she's not annoyed.

I stand in the doorway and she nudges Daddy who gets up, he doesn't say much, he makes some noises and gets my blankets
and puts them on the mattress. They just stay in their
room now, which I like.
Sometimes if my baby sister isn't awake, I climb into bed next to her and she pulls the covers back for me, and I feel a bit like a
baby myself. Everything feels right again.

Mummy asks me sometimes in the morning why I keep coming in, I don't know how to put it into words.
But just knowing she's with me makes me feel warm inside, like coming home.
A bit like solving a puzzle.
She makes the monsters go away, I don't even know how she does it. But just being next to her is enough.

So I let out a deep breath and fall asleep in safety.
Knowing these moments will become memories,
of a mattress that's always waiting.
And a mum who is too.

But just knowing she's with me makes me feel warm inside, like coming home. A bit like solving a puzzle.

THEY BLOOM BECAUSE OF YOU, JESSICA URLICHS

A Radical Love

I hope she loves herself
the way petals bloom proudly
as if they picked their outfit.

I hope she hears
the wind's orchestra
over small conversations.

I hope she knows
her echo can be loud
when she chooses silence.

I hope she finds meaning
in messy and imperfect
and dances like she knows
what to do with her hands.

I hope she feels
the warmth of the light that casts her shadow,
that's happiness I will say,
let her stay.

I hope she remembers
to enjoy her life
from deep within
so she is never without.

I hope she stares
into the mirror, wild and unapologetic,
knowing she wants this for herself,
and not just her daughters.

I hope she remembers ... so she is never without.

THEY BLOOM BECAUSE OF YOU, JESSICA URLICHS

Love Near the Chair

I vacuumed near the chair
Where the two of us would meet
From dusk till dawn, the carpet worn
From my bare and sleepy feet

Usually it would bother me
Wear and tear before my face
Hidden in plain sight
A little patch so out of place

But therein lies a story
In the quiet of those nights
A chair lived in and loved
When my embrace made things alright

The chair is mostly empty now
No early crimson skies
Seasons pressed where my feet would rest
With tired heavy eyes

We dreamed in little whispers
We lived nights like they were days
I see the proof before me
While the memories are a haze

For one day we may leave this home
We'll hand over the key
Someone will notice that thinning spot
And wonder how it came to be

We leave our mark not just in hearts
But with loving tired feet
I smile at the little spot
Where the two of us would meet.

More Than a Body

My daughter looks in the mirror,
She moves side to side,
She's seen me do the same,
Surveying my pouch where she once grew.
It's true,
It takes hard work to look a certain way,
but self-acceptance is the hardest work of all,
the long haul to rest in.
I want to tell her
that her body is the least interesting thing about her.
The way she loves, those caring hands, the way her heart shines
more than her hair.
You can make your body strong,
but it won't move the mountains you'll be remembered for.
And I want to tell her as she looks in the mirror,
that happiness
isn't shaped like a silhouette.
The edges never meet, it flows and it's free.
It

    flows   it's

        and

                free.

Heart and Hands

They say you've got your hands full
That it only gets harder from here
They say 'enjoy every minute'
As I juggle tantrums and tears
They say 'oh you'll be busy'
With a toddler at my side
A baby in my arms
'You're in for quite the ride'
My hands are full and my arms are tired
With all this weight in gold
I wonder if they miss
Those little hands they used to hold?
Because my mother's hands are empty
But every now and then
They stretch out like sunbeams
As her grandchildren fall into them
I see the look on my mother's face
And I understand after all
How blessed I am right now
To have a heart and hands so full.

Strong Women

The women in our family are young flowers and old trees
bending to the light.
The soul of each other's soul.
The blood of each other's blood.
We grow, and nurture, shelter and lift.
And when we lean on each other like dominoes,
two trees always stand nose to nose.
In case one of us falls.

My Daughter

My daughter came from me,
But she is not like me.
Instead, I wish to be like her.
Brazen and bold, fearless too.
She does not know about shrinking.
She is untamed and wild in a flawed world.
Being alive is a reason to smile,
a person passing is a reason to wave,
having a voice is a reason to shout.
She talks to everyone when we're out.
It is hard to match such unbridled joy
and so, when her outstretched hand falls,
I cheer even louder.
I sweep in and tell her
to never change.
That she is not *too much*, that the world will adjust.
I'd leap off a mountain to catch her spirit should it fall.
Maybe we're not so different after all.

Tiny Days

You walk into the kitchen, four feet tall now, you pour yourself a glass of water and it seems like the most amazing thing to me when just yesterday you were kicking the air marvelling at a mobile that danced above your head. We have conversations that leave me awestruck, but I smile and nod and drink you in and think back to postpartum when the unravelling of me took up more space than all the nappy decor. I'm not Mum yet, I'm still 'Mummy', and I still know the nape of your neck in only the way a mother could. I want to tell you that you are the most beautiful masterpiece I didn't draw. That my heart grew your heart and now you grow mine. Motherhood serves emotions with such ease, and it's quite lovely to feel such adoration on a regular afternoon. You continue to explain things with such exuberance that it makes little pockets of joy within me burst and sting. I guess it can still hurt to be forever changed in the best way.

My heart grew your heart and now you grow mine.

THEY BLOOM BECAUSE OF YOU, JESSICA URLICHS

Take Me With You

One day when you're older
You may wonder if I'm there
You might be out to lunch
Or running fingers through your hair.

You might be greeting someone new
Or hanging up the phone
Worrying, or sleeping
In company, or alone.

You might be walking down the aisle
Or saying your goodbyes
Laughing with your head flung back
A tear wiped from your eye.

You might be singing lullabies
Wishing I could hold you too
You might be cheering in a crowd
The proudest mum in the room.

And I'll be cheering with you
I'll be your happy tears
You were once a part of me
Your blood, your bones, your fears.

So, wrap your arms around yourself
Let our hearts whisper our song
A mother's love is everywhere
So you'll always take me along.

The Spaces Between

Some days I feel like I'm missing.
I'm so entangled in this season of mothering.
Planning birthday parties and forgetting how old I am. Bundling on little jackets and forgetting my own. Living ten steps ahead and still trying to remain present. I see my reflection in them more than the mirror. I see a future not so far away, where the pieces of me will return as I lose pieces of this season with it.
This season of nurturing first and often coming last.
This season of growing alongside them.
This season of being their everything.
Yes, I'm entangled in motherhood right now.
In the hard, the magic, the fleeting.

I'm entangled in motherhood right now. In the hard, the magic, the fleeting.

THEY BLOOM BECAUSE OF YOU, JESSICA URLICHS

The Vows I Didn't Write
(would read something like . . .)

We won't always see eye to eye
You're not me, and I'm not you
But when we're standing side by side,
We can see each other's view.

It won't always be an effortless love,
Though my love will be bone deep.
It burns with the stars; it will always be ours
I will love you in my sleep.

And we'll use words like they're fire
Throw blame around like knives
You'll hold my hand through tears and years
Of these beautiful little lives.

We'll collect memories like leaves
In the winter sun and summer rain
And when we're old, we'll relive the colours
As a season starts again.

We will make promises that are unspoken
We will learn what it means to choose
We'll discover the diamond in being the rock
And how rocks can also bruise.

They say that 'love' isn't enough
But when the morning is dark,
The smell of coffee and the sound of laughter echoes
Into both our hearts.

Little dimpled hands reach up
Love's longing for you and I,
And the only blue we truly know
Is the one up in the sky.

We couldn't have planned this if we tried
And I'd live this life one thousand times.

It's the simple things, the honest things
That make my heart take flight
I think this is what I would say
In the vows I didn't write.

It burns with the stars; it will always be ours I will love you in my sleep.

THEY BLOOM BECAUSE OF YOU, JESSICA URLICHS

A Mind Like Mine
(written for our neurodiverse littles)

Mummy, I know today was hard,
I'm trying to be good.
But I yelled, and cried, and got overwhelmed,
and didn't do as I should.

I know that I am different,
but I promise that I try.
The world is still quite new to me,
and I'm learning how, and why.

My head feels very noisy,
I'm distracted most of the time.
I want to move in zigzags
when I'm supposed to fall in line.

For others it seems easy,
for me it's like climbing a hill.
I want to fidget and move about
when I'm meant to be sitting still.

They tell me to be quiet,
to focus on what they ask,
but I can't hear what they're saying
when being quiet is my task.

I know you get frustrated,
when we can't get out the door.
My socks feel weird, my shoes aren't right,
I feel everything so much more.

Sometimes I wish I could change,
but I also just want to be me.
If you hold my hand, it will open your eyes
where others don't want to see.

My brain is like a busy maze,
I don't know what to do first.
There's magic in the ordinary,
my heart could simply burst.

I know that I get angry
and often make us late.
My overwhelm is big sometimes,
but my love is just as great.

I'm loyal and I'm caring,
I feel other people's pain.
I see glitter in the sunshine.
I see puddles in the rain.

My happiness can reach the sky,
I see things that others don't.
My mind wanders off a bit,
I'll ask questions others won't.

It can sometimes feel quite lonely
like no one understands,
but I feel safe with you mummy
like I can be who I truly am.

I know it seems like sometimes
I see things in black and white,
but sit with me, and you will see
that colours are oh, so bright.

Thank you for speaking up for me
and showing me it is okay.
Thank you for shining your light
when I sometimes lose my way.

I may seem like a puzzle,
but the pieces fit just fine.
It's the puzzle of the world for me
that doesn't quite align.

I often feel exhausted,
thanks for being my place to rest.
I'll always show you who I am,
you'll always get my best.

I know I don't have to tell you mum,
I know you already see . . .
Hard things can still be wonderful
and it's quite wonderful to be me.

Becoming

I will miss these little versions of the growing faces
in front of me.
I will miss the firsts and I will miss the lasts.
The last time they reach for me to pick them up, the last
mispronounced word,
the last time I (*get*) to lay with them until they fall asleep.
There is so much I will miss as they step into the next person
they're becoming,
leaving an outline of the smaller one behind.
We say goodbye to the little years much faster than we realize,
and when my heart feels heavy because of it, I remind myself of
this simple truth:
A beautiful thing happens with these goodbyes.
We welcome the incredible privilege of watching them grow.

I Mean Well

I'm not really a carefree mum,
I'm not sure it all comes so naturally.
But I mean well, you see.
I look over my shoulder,
worry about dogs running free,
I hover around you on the slide.
Someone asked me once 'What's the worst that could happen?'
'**Death**' I said, a little too fast.
She laughed. I laughed.
But I wonder what it must feel like to not see the
world with jaws,
to let them wander down to the lake, or not cut the grapes.
To not see every shelf's corner, hear every door slam
and wince for small fingers.
Worry is my runner, but love is my coach.
But the terrible comes first, because I love you so.
I just love you so.

When the World Feels Too Much

Sometimes I think about the world being terrible
and then
I think of the young boy busking outside the supermarket,
singing Coldplay,
his sweet voice in the wind
his father proud
a baby being born; coming home
an elderly couple holding hands
each time someone says,
'I saw this and thought of you'
A child's expression when they see their parent
in a crowd.
How people make art to understand the world
not for the world to understand their art
acts of kindness among strangers
a dog who waits at the door for you
how most people are good
and for all the terrible, I try to think of the happiness people still
allow into their lives
with open arms and hearts.
How people mend piece by piece,
despite all that is broken.

To Love a Boy

I loved a baby, I loved him so
And every day I'd watch him grow
The years were fast, the weeks were slow
I loved a baby, I loved him so.

I loved a toddler, I loved him so
His laugh like bubbles, cheeks like dough
Wherever I went, he too would go
I loved a toddler, I loved him so.

I loved a boy, I loved him so
Our little chats now to and fro
It goes quite fast and now I know
The baby, toddler, and boy did grow

Tick Tock went the clock.
I love them all, I love them so.

A Love That Doesn't Rest

Mum, I sit here with you now,
Each holding steaming cups
I watch you with my children
And the way their eyes light up.

Their little arms reach up to you,
You hold their heart in yours,
And I think back to those years
Of my silence and slamming doors.

I don't know if I truly said sorry,
For it pains me now to know
The love you have for your children
Only deepens as you grow.

I thought that I knew *everything*,
The way my words pierced like a knife.
The day your hand reached out
And mine stayed firmly by my side.

I was out in cars, too young for bars
I begged you to leave me be
A door between our foreheads
Crying tears neither could see.

You know I didn't mean it
All that worry I put you through
The late nights, you losing sleep
As our pathway split in two.

I didn't give you enough of my time
And if I could go back I would
I'd ask you how your day was too
I'd say more than 'fine' or 'good'.

Was it harder for you to love me then?
Did you wonder if you went wrong?
Did you grieve for where your baby went
As my heart put armour on?

Deep down I wanted to meet you halfway
Or at least somewhere close.
But I was lost as I tried to find 'here'
And I needed you there the most.

But I guess you knew this all along
Because your heart stayed on your sleeve
and love will only ever show up
if that same love never leaves.

And though the path was mine to choose
Through shadows I would roam,
You left the front light on for me
Which guided me back home.

I see you with my children now
As their head lays on your chest
I know the deepest parts of love
Because you taught me best.

A mother's love is honest
A love that doesn't rest.

The love you have for your children Only deepens as you grow.

THEY BLOOM BECAUSE OF YOU, JESSICA URLICHS

You're Doing It

I think I was too exhausted to really soak in the newborn stage.
It almost seems unfair, doesn't it.
I'll get flashes of smiles or fragments of conversations in the
evenings, it still feels a bit wispy, I wonder if it will always
be that way.
The feeling of only being half alive.
But I'm so alive, I'm right here, though I'm somewhere else too.
Somewhere in the motherhood maze.

I think back to those days often, a toddler learning to walk and
a newborn baby. The overwhelm and juggle of it. My eyes that
could leak at any moment.
The sheer state of me, a shadow in my mind, but wow
did she shine.
As do all mothers, but newborn mothers have a soft strength to
them, a loud stillness, a shy confidence.

I think back to the many moments I thought were for them,
when I held them close and rocked in our chair, I see they
were mine too.
That I needed them, my aching body pleaded for them.

I think back to the birth, the feeding, the chubby limbs, someone always on me, my husband wanting a kiss when he got home and me not wanting anyone to touch me for a second. I smile because I get it, and yet my heart twists at the thought of them needing me less.

I think back to the purees, the bottles, the mess, the many things I mastered in the kitchen with one hand. How sometimes just getting out the door was the biggest achievement, and how I had to make peace with that.

I think back to the exhaustion, trying to explain it to my husband after a hard day, but never doing it justice. The words not quite fitting in my mouth, then smiling like it didn't hurt.

I think back to the days that felt like remakes, but now I see they were all originals, especially to them. Their world expanding at a rapid rate, the most beautiful magic unfolding, did I see that?

Did I miss it through the fog?

And I think back to the days I would say,
'I just can't do this' when I was drowning.
But I was doing it.
Coming up for air, rebuilding and rising.
Maybe you'll think back like me one day,
or maybe I can remind you now.
You're doing this too.
No matter what that looks like.
You're doing it.
Because that's what mothers do.

But I was doing it. Coming up for air, rebuilding and rising.

THEY BLOOM BECAUSE OF YOU, JESSICA URLICHS

Am I Still Your Baby, Mama?

I'm only little for a little, Mama
That's what you always say
But I held my hands up to you
And you looked the other way.

Am I still your baby, Mama?
And will I be for ever?
Even though I'm not the smallest now
And it's not just us together.

Will you still hold me close to you?
Will you come to me when I call?
Will you stroke my hair as I fall asleep
Even though I'm not as small?

I'm excited and I'm curious
About this baby in our home
I miss you when you're in your room
The two of you alone.

And I'm trying to be careful, Mama
With my gentle yet clumsy hands
I know I should be patient
And I'm trying to understand.

You're really busy now
With not much time to play
I hear you cry sometimes, Mama
And I think we feel the same.

Because sometimes I feel sad
And still as happy as can be
And then people want to hold the baby
And that baby isn't me.

Though I might not be as little, Mama
You're still everything to me
You'll always be my guiding star
No matter how big I seem.

Then I lifted my hands to you
And you scooped me up in your arms
I softened, just like I always do
Our special kind of calm.

And it was just us again
Even though so much had changed
You whispered, as we swayed together
That your love for me was the same.

And then the little cries came
But you kept your hand in mine
And you cradled us together
As you sang 'you are my sunshine'.

And I realized in that moment
That it is still me and you,
And now I have the gift
Of being a sister too.

And Mama, then you whispered to me
In our new and special mould,
'You'll always be my baby,
Just heavier to hold.'

My Middle Child

Maybe right now, darling
You feel a bit between
A little in the middle
A tiny bit unseen.

You've always been the youngest
You've looked up to your brother
And now when you look down
There's suddenly another.

Here's what you need to know, my love
Although we're rearranged
You may not be the smallest
But my love for you hasn't changed.

You've grown up overnight it seems
It's hard on you, I know
You may have to curl to fit on my lap
But these arms you won't outgrow.

I remember it like yesterday
The moment I first saw you
I fell headfirst, for a second time
With a confidence so new.

It was you, my love, that gave me
A patience, and a roar
Motherhood took her hand in mine
Differently than before.

Life was busy, slow and fast
It was hard juggling you two
And now we have another
I know I can do it, because of you.

So let me pick you up again
In the only way we mould
My darling, I'll always carry you
For that you are never too old.

It's such a special role, you see
That not just anyone could do
For you are a big sister now
Someone looks up to you.

Watching you together
It makes my heart just burst
They may call you the middle child
But to me, you all come first.

The Friends We Hold Close

We often romanticize lovers and fate,
but what of the women who show up at our gate?
When the lock is firm and the hinge is broken;
they hear your silence, and don't wait for the open.
They look past the weeds, they bring heart and home
their flaws, and their truths,
what a thing to be known.
We show up for these friends
in the summer and the blue
There's no one else I have to be than me when I'm with you.
And we give them our lives, our laughter, our pain,
we promise them time to the very last train.
My daughter will know of the ones I keep near
and how a love story begins right here.

This Hard Has Been My Happiest

I could talk about all the ways a third child means you're outnumbered, how the juggle of your heart, mind and mental load only leaves room for quick-fire decisions, an exhaustion you never knew.

I could talk about how the giving never feels like enough, someone is always needing, someone is usually crying or yelling (sometimes over the baby's head). They know you're only one person, and yet they're too young to comprehend that.

I could talk about the overuse of the bouncer, the naps in the carrier, and how life suddenly feels like a tornado whirling around you while you're stuck in slow motion.

But I could also talk about how the world doesn't implode when things are forgotten and how maybe I needed that reminder, that things being a little more up in the air has simultaneously grounded me.

I could talk about my lack of confidence to take all three on outings alone just yet. How it's meant a lot of togetherness at home instead. But laughter fills the yard and memories are still being made. The simplicity is settling.

I could talk about the night wakes being easier. Not just because I'm used to it, but because they're our moments. She's not feeding wide-eyed with screaming and chaos around her. It's just us in the quiet of my future best memories.

I could talk about how my body has changed the most this time around, but also how I'm comfortable in my new size. It still feels a bit foreign, but my body has given me a lot.

I could talk about how fast this is going, and this time it really is. She's rolling over now, but I'm not fixated on milestones this time. It's taken two for me to realize I don't need to rush moments through, time will do that for me.

I could talk about her room being unfinished, her clothes being mismatched, and how she gets a little more floor time than I would like, but then she flashes me that just-woken-up smile and none of it matters.

I know I can't be everything to everyone, all at one time. But this third time? It's given me the grace to accept I don't have to be, and I'm a better version of myself because of it.

> This hard has been my happiest.
> So I guess I could talk about that.

Who She Would Have Been

I have children now, so I can never be sure as to who I would have been without them.
But I'm entirely sure it would have been someone different.
She would have found her way, faced her demons, grown into herself eventually.
But the one with children, this version of me, she has learnt to do these things in times she felt she could give nothing, while being someone's everything.
She found her way as she was guiding little feet.
She faced her demons in the hopes they wouldn't have to, and she grew into herself as she grew someone else.
Not just her child, but a new version of herself.
I can never be entirely sure of who I would have been,
but I've never been more sure
of where I'm meant to be.

She grew into herself as she grew someone else.

THEY BLOOM BECAUSE OF YOU, JESSICA URLICHS

When Mummy Was Your Name

The baby is crying,
it's 5 a.m., and time to start the day.
Everything aches, it's dark outside,
and the kids want you to play.

Lunchboxes to take, appointments to make,
you'll remember, or you won't.
You'll hold the baby in your arms,
until one day you don't.

The kids are fighting, your head's a mess,
the house is never clean.
Computer is next to the baby monitor,
you're working with two screens.

You're fuelling little bodies,
while food goes flying from afar.
You'll wish that things were easier
and then one day they are.

Your body creaks like floorboards,
someone always needs you now.
You're torn in all directions
as the day comes crashing down.

Cushioned bums, and full round tums
stains all down your top.
At night you hear them call your name
and one day it will stop.

Fingerprints, and perfect hands,
a house that is a home.
Sloppy kisses, knotty hair,
growing, growing, grown.

Grubby faces, muddy shoes.
Beauty and bittersweet.
You are the star of their show,
and soon you'll pull up a seat.

These exhausting little days are long
and this is how it goes.
It's messy, loud and full of love,
as fast as it is slow.

You wish for things to hurry up,
and also stay the same.
You hold on to these moments,
and also wish for change.

And look back, like all mothers do,
when 'Mummy' was your name.

First Day

There's a thousand ways **I love you**, but here are just a few.
I will pack your lunch with the things you **love**,
and I will think of **you**.
I look at you in your uniform, so big on your **love**ly frame,
and underneath your collar, I have carefully written **you**r name.
I have labelled all your things, my **love**,
and I have packed **your** bag to go,
I would **love** a photo of you first before **you** go and grow.
I hope you laugh and make some friends, sweet **love**, I hope they're kind.
I'll say goodbye and wave at the gate, but **you** will be
on my mind.
It's part of our story, mostly yours, this chapter that is new.
I will let my heart go, and I **love** to think of the wonderful
things **you** will do.
I'll be there when the bell rings, as true as the sky is blue.
Tell me all about your day.
I love you, I love you, I love you.

Be Seeing You

Goodbye you say
Such a little word
Too small for all it means
It's you after all
Who takes the place
Of the you that suddenly leaves.

Goodbye you say
The babbling you,
Crawling you, and then
Pointing, laughing,
Running you
Pass the baton again.

And it's not a given
These chapters we live in
This thing that we call time
So I'm grateful, I am
Even as your hand
Slowly lets go of mine.

I'm not really sad
It's you after all
And I don't want to dwell
But for such a great love
It seems unfair
I can't give them all a farewell.

Because rocks are still treasures
Before they shine
Feet are for jumping
And trees are to climb
Joy always finds you
In such simple ways
And it's all just to say
I am loving these days . . .

So stay a bit longer
Don't go too soon
But even if you do
How lucky am I
To love the you then
And to always love the now you.

I'll say hello as you wave goodbye
I'll keep all of you in my dreams
Goodbye is such a little word
Too small for all it means.

Goodbye is such a little word
Too small for all it means.

THEY BLOOM BECAUSE OF YOU, JESSICA URLICHS

There's Something About That Third Child

She is all the things I felt for my first and second,
but slowed down.

She is all the milestones I have witnessed before,
that I am not rushing.

She is all the long days that I have lived,
that I am holding on to.

She is all the sleepless nights that are still hard,
but it's just our time, and there's not a lot of that any more.

She is all the moments I am reliving,
and yet they are so completely different.

She is all the love that lifts the corners of her siblings' mouths
just at the sight of her.

She is everything that I didn't know I needed.
Because there's just something about that third child.

The Mental Load

The mental load is one of the hardest things about motherhood.
Because it's invisible, because it's expected, and necessary.
Because it's silent on the outside, and sirens on the inside.
It's like constant project management. Sometimes menial,
largely momentous.
Often heavy, mostly hidden.
Sorting, arranging, organizing, balancing, planning,
preparing, anticipating.
Remembering, remembering, *remembering*.
It's like having 200 tabs open in your brain at any given time and
switching off might mean losing them all.
It's like watching a movie play out in front of you with someone
talking the whole way through.
Sometimes we just want someone else to make the lists, make
the decisions, know what comes next.

It's not the doing that's exhausting, it's the thinking for everyone.
It might be invisible,
but it leaves visible cracks.
It leaves no room for us to be in the moment.
It leaves no room for ourselves.

Because it's silent on the outside, and sirens on the inside.

THEY BLOOM BECAUSE OF YOU, JESSICA URLICHS

The Mums Who Walk Each Other Home

Mum friendships are like another language.
When they lend an ear with their own chaos in the background.
'I see you'
When they give you their time, though there is little to spare.
'I'm here for you'
When they offer their help even when they're drowning too.
'I'm with you'

Each act of kindness more like a love note.
'You can trust me with the most vulnerable parts of your life' they smile,
as they shuffle through your door.

Cracked Open

Having children has left me more exposed
and vulnerable than ever before, and yet
despite that, I care so much less about what
people think of me.
It's like motherhood has broken me,
healed me, and humbled me all at once.

Rested Eyes

I don't want to go through postpartum again.
I know I am at capacity physically and emotionally with the children we have.
I don't want to add to my family, I now want to focus on raising them.
And yet...
The strange sadness I feel that I will never be pregnant again, to watch my tummy ripple at nighttime with little elbows and knees, never whisper through tears as their eyes focus on mine, 'hello sweetheart, I'm your mummy'.
Our last baby is just about to start walking. Another new version to welcome, another one to farewell. The joy and complete feeling is overwhelming, and the wistful feeling lingers with it.
If only I could visit each little version of them whenever I felt like it, not just in my heart, but hold those little dimpled hands for ever.
Study their face a bit longer with rested eyes. Eyes that have seen the beautiful chaos.
I don't want another baby.
But I don't want to forget.
Maybe that's what I'm feeling.

I don't want another baby. But I don't want to forget.

THEY BLOOM BECAUSE OF YOU, JESSICA URLICHS

Missing: Brain

I left my brain somewhere in the house I think,
tucked away in the unmade sheets,
maybe it's by the to-do list or in the beeping washing machine.
I might have left it at the grocery store or in the tower of bowls
of swimming cereal,
or it's in the car with the empty tank of fuel.
Or the emails I need to unsubscribe from but it's so much faster
to delete them.
I'd say it's in the abyss, with that word I'm trying to find,
I know it,
what is it?
IRONY.
I've checked the drawers of clothes that need upsizing
and I've looked through the overgrown garden,
hoping for a glimmer like a lost earring.
It's probably in the past or future,
hoping one day it will show up in the present.
Or maybe it's still between the lines of that article,
hiding under guilt from forgotten anniversaries, appointments,
myself, yes I've forgotten myself a bit.
It should show up soon, this is embarrassing.
Or perhaps momentarily it went away, the second my heart had
more to say.
I don't think so though,
it's a nice thought anyway.

A Love Note to My Younger Self

You know I wouldn't be where I am
if it weren't for you.
I know that sounds dramatic,
but I promise, it is true.

I wouldn't have fought the storms,
the ones that tore me apart.
I wouldn't have pieced myself back together
if it weren't for your heart.

And all those times you cried
in the shadows where you sat.
There is so much light coming,
I just want to tell you that.

And the times that you were hurt,
where it felt too hard to cope;
you didn't know it then,
but you always held out hope.

You've been let down a bit,
looked for home in ruins and rubble,
and you've made a lot of mistakes,
got yourself in a bit of trouble.

Not everything was meant for you,
and love would sometimes leave,
but it gave you space to bloom,
to see the forest for the trees.

You grew through the cracks anyway,
you would always find the sun.
Your feet were heavy, but they moved,
and I watched you become.

So let's go on a journey,
come on, let's get in the car.
There will be a few wrong turns,
but it's really not that far.

And maybe you will turn to me
and ask if you can stay,
and I'll shake my head because we know
it doesn't work that way.

Because we're so different now,
a whole lifetime ago.
As I take you past the places,
the ones I used to know.

I'll tell you, 'it ends up OK'
if only then you knew.
My brave and strong younger self,
I'm really proud of you.

There is so much light coming, I just want to tell you that.

THEY BLOOM BECAUSE OF YOU, JESSICA URLICHS

Why Are You So Tired?

I would say
It's the nighttime theatre
Of musical pillows
But really –
It's the day.
When my head is
Filled with so many minds
A stream of hopes
A galaxy of dreams
A tipped-over bin of questions
That even at night
It's never quiet.

But We Lived

We didn't do a lot today
The sun was shining so we sat outside,
ate some lunch,
hung the washing.
My daughter pointed to a plane while she held up pegs.
Sat under a tree, played with the sprays of the hose while I tried
to water plants.
I didn't get to it all, there's always so much to do,
so much, but we spent some time.
Some days we need to do less so we can *be* more.
Let go of the weight of responsibility on our chest for a
moment so we can remember what it's like to *live*.
We got tricked along the way.
But my children remind me of the irony,
of how we believe that life can only be enjoyed
when it's all done.

I Miss You

The cries continue from the back seat, each one pierces my heart deeper, each one adds five minutes to our journey. It's only moments before we turn on each other because, how can you be so calm? And why am I so stressed?
Drive faster.
Slow down.
I miss you.

We go to bed at different times, but our shadows grow long together at night. We take turns wandering down the hallway, we compare who needs sleep the most, who needs a shower the most.
I'm tired.
We're tired.
I miss you.

Look at the baby, see the curls, I catch your eye and together we smile. The inventory of the day swirls in my head and remembering to hug you is buried under it all.
I've never felt more me, and yet so incredibly different.
It's us.
It's still us.
I miss you.

Celebrate the firsts, feel heavy over the lasts, smile at strangers at the café when the babbling begins, smile in the photos, smile but remember the blue, remember the fire I spat, the forgotten kisses.
A leave of absence.
A slow return.
I miss you.

We laugh in the day, stay up at night nursing temperatures and sickness, I say goodbye to you in my dressing gown, screenshot more recipes I probably won't make. We have never loved so hard as 'Mum' or 'Dad'.
It suits you, it suits us.
But why did no one tell us,
I'd miss you.

There isn't much time for each other, there are still no lavish gestures, just small offerings of morning coffee, playing you a new song I know you will like. You take the monitor, I take your hand. How have we grown so strong in this fragile season?
I should tell you, this is enough right now. It has to be.
You hold me.
You know me.
I love you.

A leave of absence.
A slow return.
I miss you.

THEY BLOOM BECAUSE OF YOU, JESSICA URLICHS

Tiptoe, Off You Grow

Tiptoe, off you grow,
Wobbly legs, away they go
They're happy tears, don't you know.

Last baby, first teeth
Hold you close, next to me
Little body, watch you breathe.

Nursing chair, tired bliss
Hold your foot, give it a kiss
A little moment, one I'll miss.

Scoop you up, little star
Your only view, where we are
Nape of your neck, now afar.

Little shadow, sleeps alone
Chatting, waving, bigger clothes
Holds my cheek, nose to nose.

Happy tears, off you grow
Wobbly legs, away you go.

The School Gate

Truthfully, I wish I was better
At prattling on about the weather
About the kids and what they're learning
Like nothing else inside is burning.

Here all I am is someone's mum
A five-minute window to talk like one
The questions are short, the answers are shorter.
Chats are vanilla, as thin as water.

But I smile along, and I try my best
But my problem is this, I cannot say less.
My words are clipped, my mind's on the run
And I know you are more than 'so and so's mum'.

I want your storms, not weather chat
Give me all of the details, I'm better with that.
Your humour, home life, rebellion, grit
And I know it's my fault that my small talk is shit.

I don't know how to give
Just a little bit.

I want your storms, not weather chat Give me all of the details, I'm better with that.

THEY BLOOM BECAUSE OF YOU, JESSICA URLICHS

Today You Turn Six

Six years ago
To this very day
You came into this world
And everything changed

The glittery nights
The rivers; sky blue
They still held their beauty
But I marvelled at you

It has gone by so fast
From the moment we met
You won't remember
What I can't forget

The soft dimpled hands
How you fell in my arms
How your bottom lip dropped
My heartbeat, your calm

And I look at you now
And my heart bursts with pride
As I watch you be brave
And curious, and kind

Your opinions are forming
Your personality shines
To raise someone who sparkles
Means I cannot dim mine

So thank you for this privilege
Of watching you grow
You're a wonderful little soul
That I'm so proud to know

We now read books together
And when I turn out the light
You tell me small stories
In the quiet of the night

But your story is my favourite
With so much yet untold
Happy birthday to you
My big six-year-old.

For Grandad

The puzzle pieces are scattered.
Memories bruised; thoughts lost.
But sometimes they open like a rose, and I see you
for a moment,
And then the petals fall.
I hope you know you belong.
I hope you know I see you for all you were.
I will tell my children about you as they grow.
Because even though you don't remember me,
When you looked at her today
I saw it tear through you,
The most precious memory of all,
Love.

I Point Out Every Blossom Tree

Sometimes it's the little things:
The moonlight across their ceramic skin
When someone offers you a coffee
How the morning sun spills through your window
Driving around a bit longer to finish your favourite song
A poem that unlocks you
A line you can't stop reading
The familiar scent of closeness
Brand-new baby leaves
Or a blossom-tree-lined street
The calm smell of an old book
A little hand in yours.

Stay close to it all,
all there is to love,
as endless as the sky.

A Human First

They said it gets easier
In some ways they were right
But I still can't separate mother and wife
I still can't pull apart days from nights.

I find that I still struggle
Watch myself from above
The mother who plays make-believe,
To the wife who makes love.

In the evenings I soothe,
Sing a lullaby song
My hair, her comfort,
So I keep it long.

Make appointments, make time,
Make do, make beds
I still gather myself
To unravel instead.

I still wish away moments,
Then long for their stay
Collect memories like treasures
And guilt like small graves.

I still feel the weight
Of a world that's unkind
Still say the wrong thing,
Still get stuck in my mind.

Daydream in the car,
Feel joy creep in
Wonder how I arrived
Wonder where I begin.

Tiny hands like feathers
Obligations like stones
It strengthens, and hardens
And grows in my bones.

I still welcome small footsteps
As floorboards creak
Press my face to the pillow
Feel the salt on my cheek.

I still feel a rage
That burns on my tongue
And at night when the moon
Swaps shifts with the sun

I still make plans
I still hold hands
Still pick through the days
Like grains of sand.

I'm still learning how to live
With this love and fear
I kiss their head,
Their scent – my air.

They said it gets easier
But I wonder which part?
I never healed from the birth
When they pulled out my heart.

I see it before me
I watch it burst
A mother, a wife,
A human first.

You'll Always Be With Me

My son lets out a little sob,
because he doesn't want me to die.
It's come out of nowhere, and everywhere,
as the day turns into night.

His lashes long, eyes like jewels,
shining with his tears.
I wonder what I can possibly say
to help calm his fears.

I think of how hard today has been
as we lay and I stroke his head.
I can't count the sorrys on my hand
so I count the stars instead.

I tell him I'm not going anywhere.
I tell him I love him too.
I don't tell him the thought of us being apart
rips my sky in two.

And somehow, I am filled with guilt
to be loved this close to the bone.
He sees all of me imperfectly
and still reaches for me like home.

And yet here we are in this uncertain world,
more certain than ever before –
that without each other, nothing makes sense.
Like two feet without a floor.

That is the weight of a love so big
the kind that aches within.
You mourn the versions been and gone –
miss moments you're still in.

I want to tell him I'll always be here,
though I know this isn't true.
I don't say 'you'll always walk with me,
but I won't always walk with you'.

I tell him he has my heart, always.
Even when it departs this place.
I tell him in every universe
I will always see his face.

There's a version of us in every life
and all the versions you'll be
even when I'm at one with the wind,
the shining stars, and the sea.

I whisper, 'in every life of mine
you will always be with me.'

The Current

We are tiny boats on a rough sea
So we must stop worrying about all the things we said or
didn't say,
did or didn't do.
Our child's tears, or our mistakes.
We're all unfinished, unpolished, and that's the best part.
We must stop looking so far into the future for the relief of
calm waters.
Grow with them, and show up.
Be tender and true, love yourself too.
One day when they hold their child's cheeks they may see their
mother's hands,
older and open.
A wild sea tracing their face like the calmest waters.
Always exactly where you were meant to be.

Where Love Lives

If you ever wonder
How much you mean to me
My love is far too big
For all the sky, and all the sea
Too big for every twinkling star,
The rolling hills and moon
The universe itself would burst
With all my love for you
And though you cannot see it
It lives somewhere quite close
When your head lays on my chest
You'll hear it there the most
Even though this great big love
Could move mountains apart
It fits somewhere quite small
It's found in both our hearts.

*My love is far
too big
For all the sky,
and all the sea.*

THEY BLOOM BECAUSE OF YOU, JESSICA URLICHS

Boys Will Be Boys

When they say 'boys will be boys'
I hope they don't just mean tiny tornadoes
and thunderous feet.
My son is also the soft glow of the moon,
with tender temples beneath my kiss.
He radiates yellow –
like the blooms he notices on our walks,
golden honey, slouching butter in the sun.
He whispers 'I love you',
holds my hand
tender and steady.
He shares gentle thoughts
from under his scruffy hair.
And yes, he is loud,
but watch how he uses that same voice to care.
His heart is unguarded, mine is rewritten.
Yes, boys will be boys.
And aren't they wonderful.

When I Tell My Daughter 'I Love You Too'

When my daughter tells me she loves me
I want to reply I am not me without her,
that only *with* her, I am.
We are made of each other
for each other,
and the word 'love' will never be big enough to describe
the heart of my heart,
or love's own longing.
How she has coloured me in,
at the sight of her; poetry.
How I will find her in every universe
just as she finds me in my dreams.
How this love will never boast or take, but simply offer itself
endlessly.
Because my heart doesn't just beat for her.
It beats because of her.
She is love.

I will find her in every universe just as she finds me in my dreams.

THEY BLOOM BECAUSE OF YOU, JESSICA URLICHS

The Song of Motherhood

We're in the season of chaos
and later on we'll see
that all those notes, high and low
made a melody.

We're in the season of tired
colour, mess, and toys
those separate notes that fill our days
sound more like one big noise.

We're in the season of togetherness
fatigued, loved-up, and loud
entwined in exhausting intimacy
and never being more proud.

We're in the season of emotions
holding them like treasure
wearing every single mood
trying to predict the weather.

We're in the season of 2 a.m. feeds
school pick-ups, and fairy wings
juggling work, with nights like days
surrendering to all it brings.

We're in the season of fragments
wondering will it be for ever?
They take your heart wherever they go
so you never feel put together.

We're in the season of constant
a mind ticking and brewing
remember when you were a human being
before a human doing?

We're in the season of growth
of a time that's suddenly been
watching their beautiful bloom
and also wishing for evergreen.

We're in the season of loving
and loving how they love too
the exquisite way you mould to them
how nothing's felt more true.

The season of leaning into your voice
and blocking out all the 'shoulds'
fast and slow, high and low
the song of motherhood.

Not Just the Family Dog
(for the dogs that see us through motherhood)

You're more than just a dog
And so much more than just a pet
You became our family
From the moment that we met.

And whatever happened, big or small
There was always you
I guess I never realized
Just how much you'd see me through.

Big paws that you grew into
And a tail that never stopped
We'd laze about the lawn
With a ball you'd never drop.

I hated to say goodbye
I'd leave you something to gnaw
Then come home to a confetti
Of toilet paper on the floor.

But we made a pact, you and I
Though I hated to leave you alone
You loved me just for being
And I promised I'd always come home.

You saw us on our wedding day
And you grew fast like dogs do
And one day I fell pregnant
And somehow, you just knew.

You always trailed behind me
Always close, never apart
And then I placed him close to you
As you met my beating heart.

Your sniffing nose lay on his lap
A forever bond exchanged
And it saddens me somewhat to think
That this is where it changed.

You saw me up all hours at night
Your eyes big with concern
The noises new, our moods had changed
And you too, had to learn.

Then the post arrived at nap time
You barked, and I felt rage
I called you 'the dog' for the first time then
Which was maybe the hardest stage.

You saw me in my baby blues
My worry and my doubt
You came with me on that first walk
When the sun had just come out.

And we'd pound the pavements every day
Back to you and me
With baby decor all over the floor
And our little family.

And over the years we added two
Each baby you'd adore
It got so busy that there were times
I forgot to pat you at the door.

I'd grab the keys, sort the bags
And yell 'have you got your shoes?'
And in a flurry the door clicked shut
I forgot to say bye to you.

I know you're getting older now
I'm seeing lots more greys
I'll try to slow down a little bit
And I'm sorry for those days.

I watch you with the kids in the yard
In the golden hour bliss
Racing around, tongue hanging out
It's hard to imagine life before this.

But you've been there from the beginning
Right from the very start
Always loving, and forgiving.
My first baby, my first heart.

I still think of those trembling legs
As you'd eat your food with joy
Your too-big bowl, now with a chip,
Each baby's favourite toy.

And in every photo on my phone
There's a tail, or blur of hair
Especially if the kids are eating
You're in the frame somewhere.

You've seen us through a lot
And some days have been rough
I know we have longer together
But it will never be enough.

You've loved us all, no questions
And simply because I'm me
You're not the family dog
But a dog that is family.

Three Plus Me

I'm walking three paths at once, four if you count my own.
One minute you come to this fork in the road, and instead of
choosing between them, they coexist alongside each other.
They tangle and eventually veer off in different directions and
somehow you all come back together, like you never let
go of their hand.

I'm watching three paintings come to life, four if you
count my own.
Sometimes I think back to who I was, a million years ago. I
have taken strokes of her with me, the soul of her. I have shed
uncertainty and doubt, I have let them scribble all over me,
breathe new colour into me. I have become gentler with myself,
the moment I was framed by them.

I'm reading three stories at once, four if you count my own.
Pages unnumbered, coming back to chapters, underlining
memories, and suddenly watching words appear on pages before
me. Little hands holding pencils, writing their own endings, so
many endings, so many more beginnings, with me, their co-
author, for now.

I have three little shadows, four if you count my own.
They hop and skip and climb up walls with the sun. I move,
they follow, I follow where they move. How beautiful to know a
shadow in the way you know a scent, a smile, love.

I have three little hearts, one if you count my own.
They live within mine, they fill me with that terrifying kind of
love, the one that only a parent can know, the kind that makes
your heart beat faster, explode, and steady. The kind that keeps
beating for ever. A love so big it has nowhere to go,
but everywhere.

The Good Old Days

Now that you're a mother
They say that you will change
And what a gift it is
To never be the same
To take with you the old
And rearrange the new
To hold a little hand
That grows alongside you
You'll hope you don't forget
You'll try to remember 'then'
You'll drift back to the 'good old days'
Seeing now, that this, was them.

You'll drift back to the 'good old days' Seeing now, that this, was them.

THEY BLOOM BECAUSE OF YOU, JESSICA URLICHS

Today You Turn Seven

You're no longer six
And you're not quite yet eight
Today you turn seven
Your favourite date.

I bet you didn't know
That it's one of mine too.
For today is the day
That I first met you.

It's all pretty quick now
Off, off we go,
Adventures are waiting
No time to go slow!

A foot out the door
Always places to be
It's you and the world
And less you and me.

But if you could pick one
You'd always choose home
It will always be here
Even when you are grown.

You've got your own friends
Your own sayings now too
You're getting so tall
And my love grows with you.

You still hold my hand
Our chats make me smile
Questions an inch
Your thoughts are a mile.

But life's not a race
So, let's take it steady
Life lessons are coming
I can see them already.

And I'll always be here
Even if you should fall
All those tiny days
Were quite big after all.

For they got us here
My own pot of gold
Happy birthday to you
My seven-year-old.

Your Motherhood Lives On

A mother sows seeds for a forest she will never see. Long after she leaves, the blooms will stretch into gardens, and the trees will strengthen and grow. The ripples she made will be the whisper of a thought or memory. She leaves behind her love, her touch, her time. She leaves behind her motherhood in the warmth that shines in others. On and on, long after she is gone.

Here We Are

Here we are until we aren't
when sleep is but a dream
the seasons promise us of change
much further than it seems

Here we are until we aren't
the switch beside my bed
the glow of light upon your face
your little resting head

Here we are until we aren't
while I am still your warmth
my morning view, a promise of
how sun shines after storms

Here we are until we aren't
strength, surrender, tears
rocking, loving, soothing, humming
for what has now been years

And though I've tried to rush this season
something in me can't
So right now
here we are
until, of course, we aren't.

They Bloom Because of You

You can't do all the things
And I'm not saying not to try
But in this season of thriving here
Over there might look a bit dry.

You can't give yourself to everything
You can't pour from an empty cup
It's hard to get the to-do list down
With little hands reaching up.

I know that you've been scrolling
Seeing deep cleaning, and fancy meals
And kids dressed in matching outfits
Their rooms with aesthetic feels.

But I haven't had time to wash my sheets
There are weeds all through the yard
I'm trying to get some work done
And in this season it's really hard.

So I think we need to normalize
While you're helping small ones grow
That this is important work too
And you might not think it shows.

But if I walked into your home right now
With mess all over the floor
A baby bouncing on your hip
And rubbish at the door

I'd feel completely welcome
And know I wasn't alone
Mothering isn't housekeeping
It's not what makes a house a home.

It isn't juggling all the things
It's a constant start and stop
Forgetting, remembering, overwhelm
It's knowing which balls we can drop.

So I see you in the unseen
In this season and what it brings
Being superwoman does not mean
Doing all the things.

It's okay for weeds to grow
Around all the things you do
Focus on the flowers:
They bloom because of you.

Focus on the flowers: They bloom because of you.

THEY BLOOM BECAUSE OF YOU, JESSICA URLICHS

Acknowledgements

To the editors at Penguin, thank you for helping to bring this collection to life with such care and love, allowing my poems to be seen and treasured across the world.

To all the mothers, my own mother, and my nana – who still pauses to read every new poem that appears online – thank you.

To every reader, whatever season you're in, every time you say 'same', every story you share, you're helping heal something, somewhere. Your support has made all of this possible.

And most of all, to my children. Without your love, and lessons, these pages would be empty.